ANATOMY Coloring Book

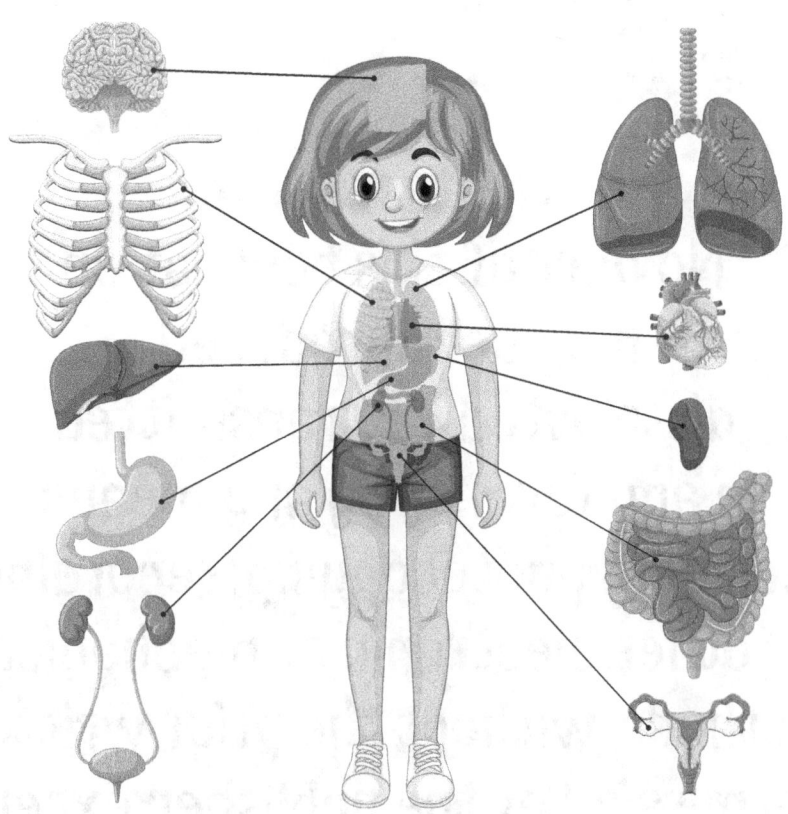

This Book Belongs To

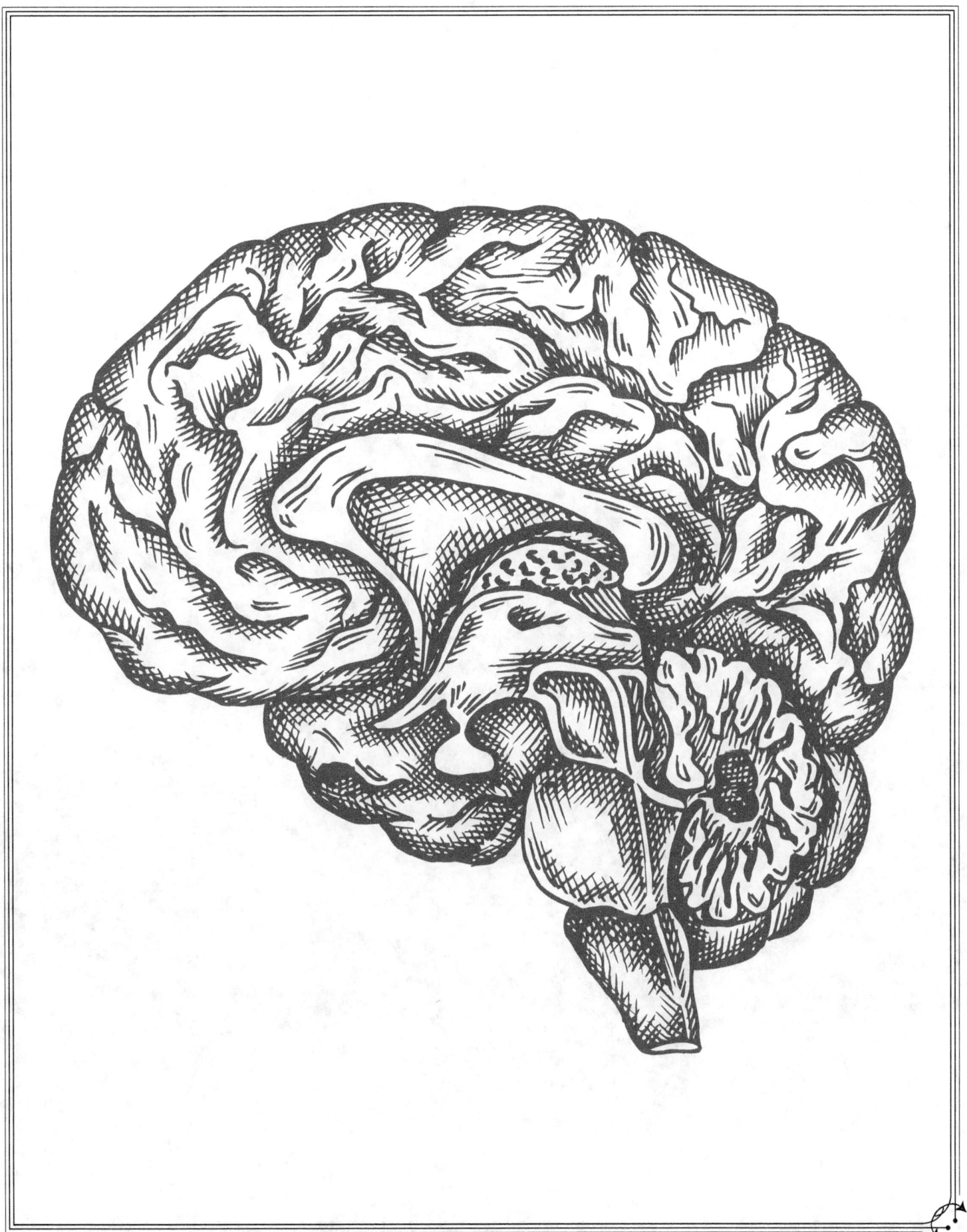

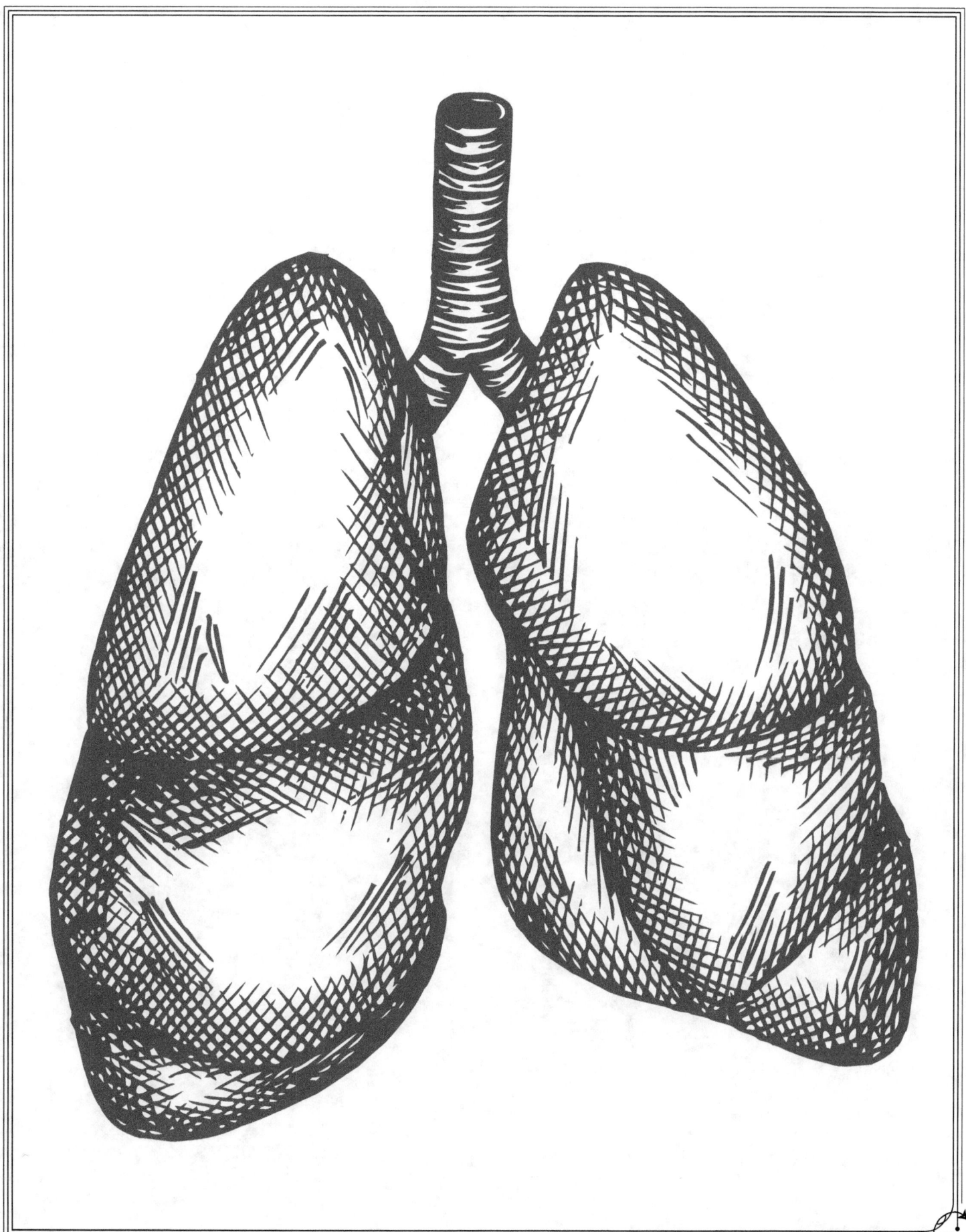

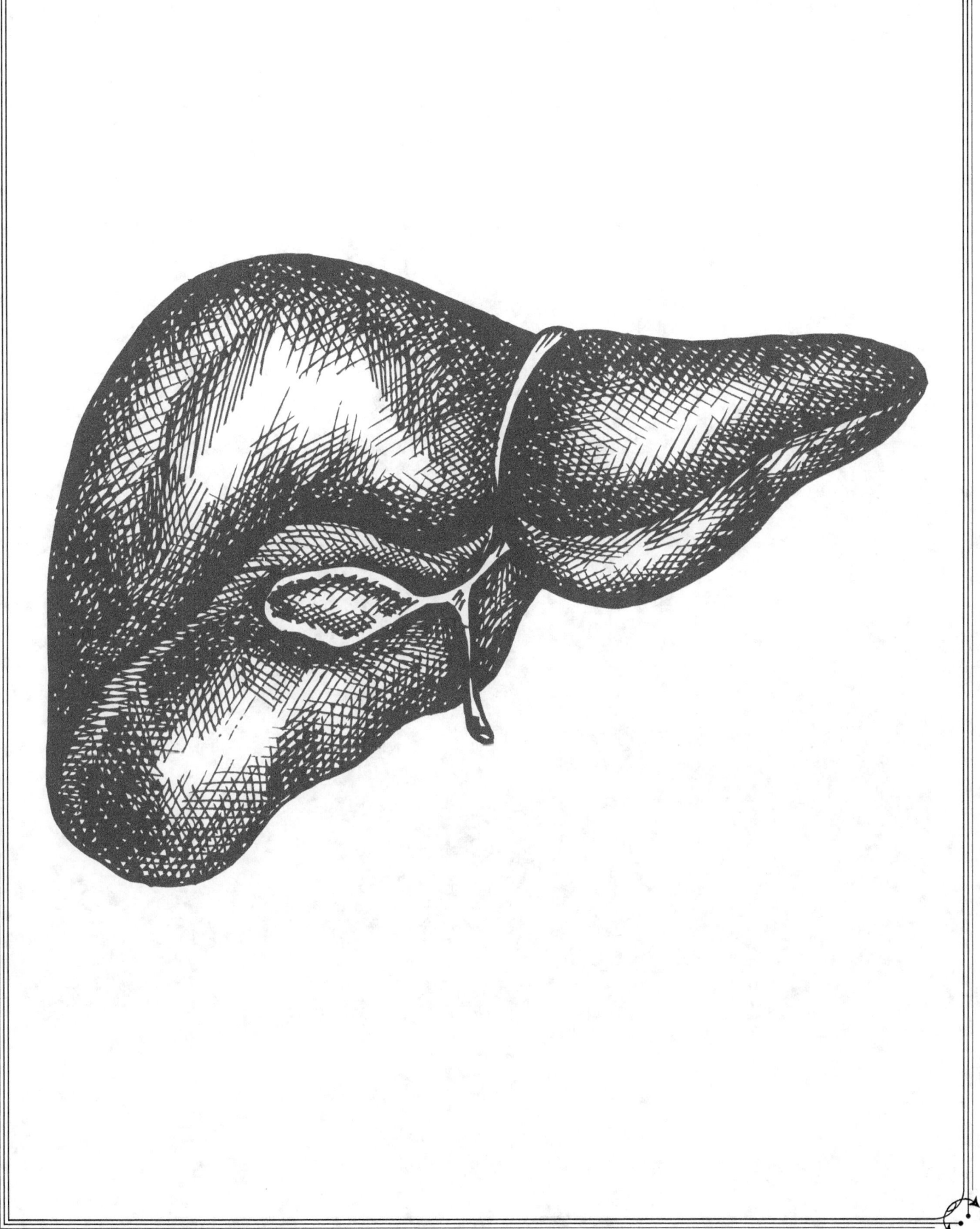

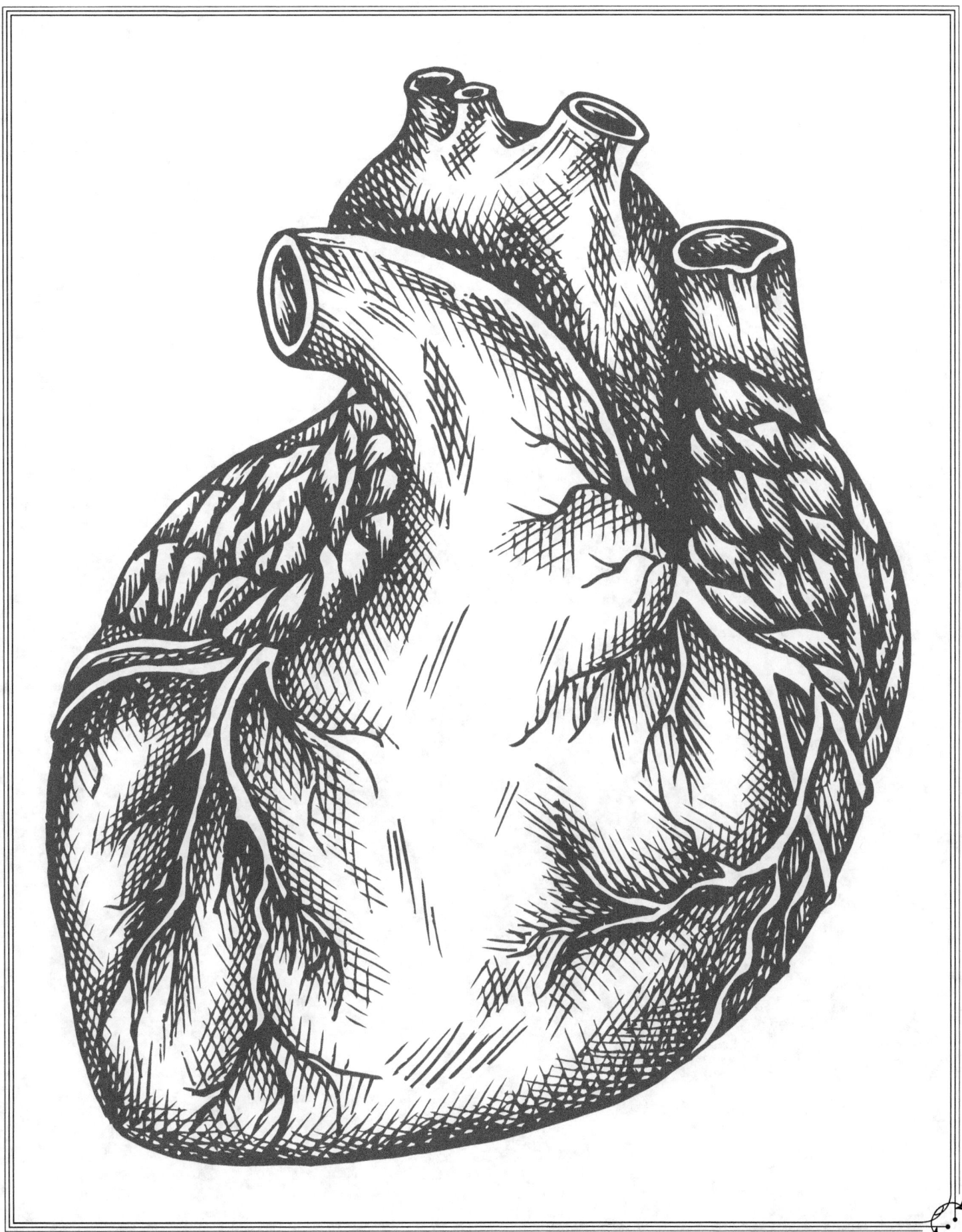

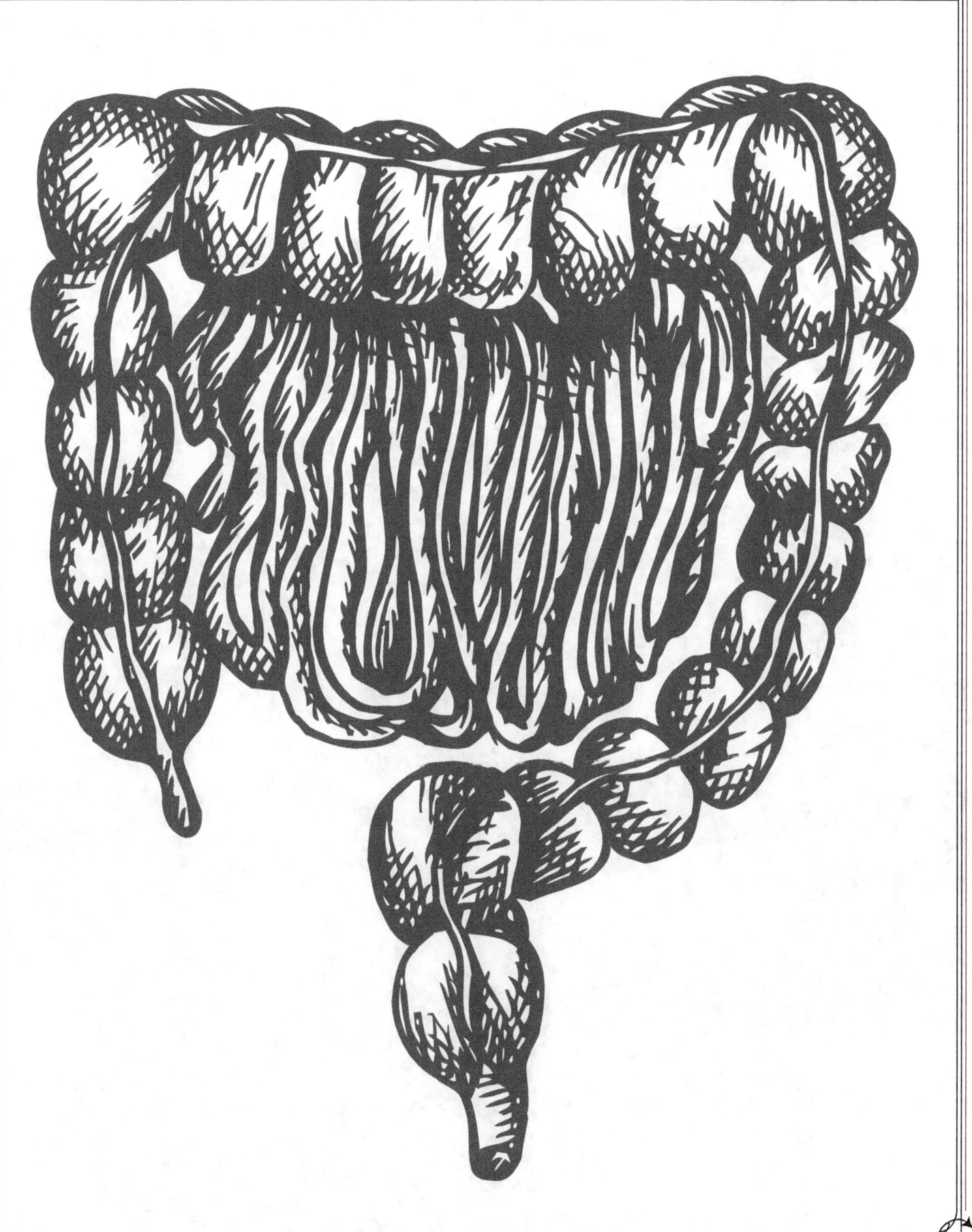

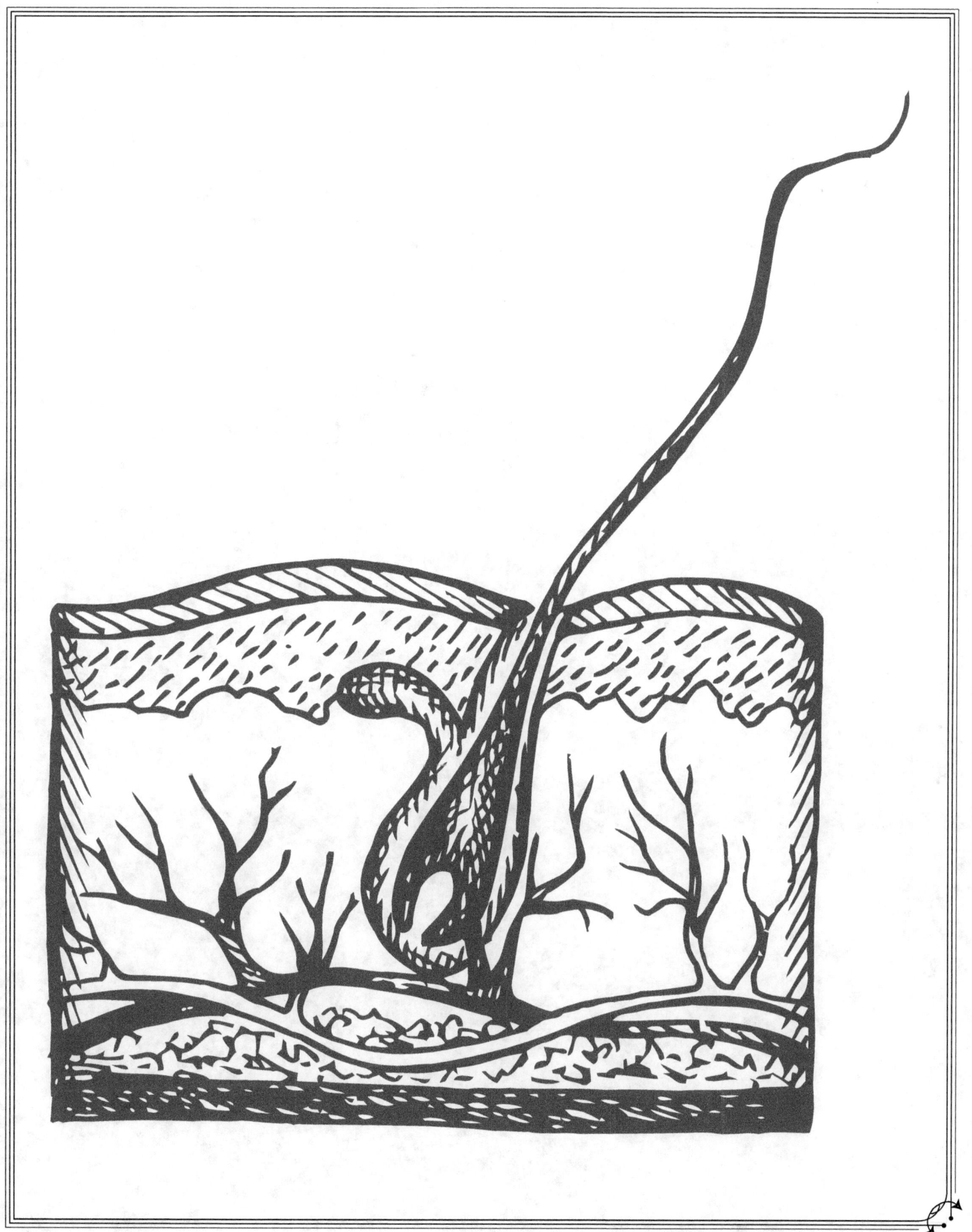

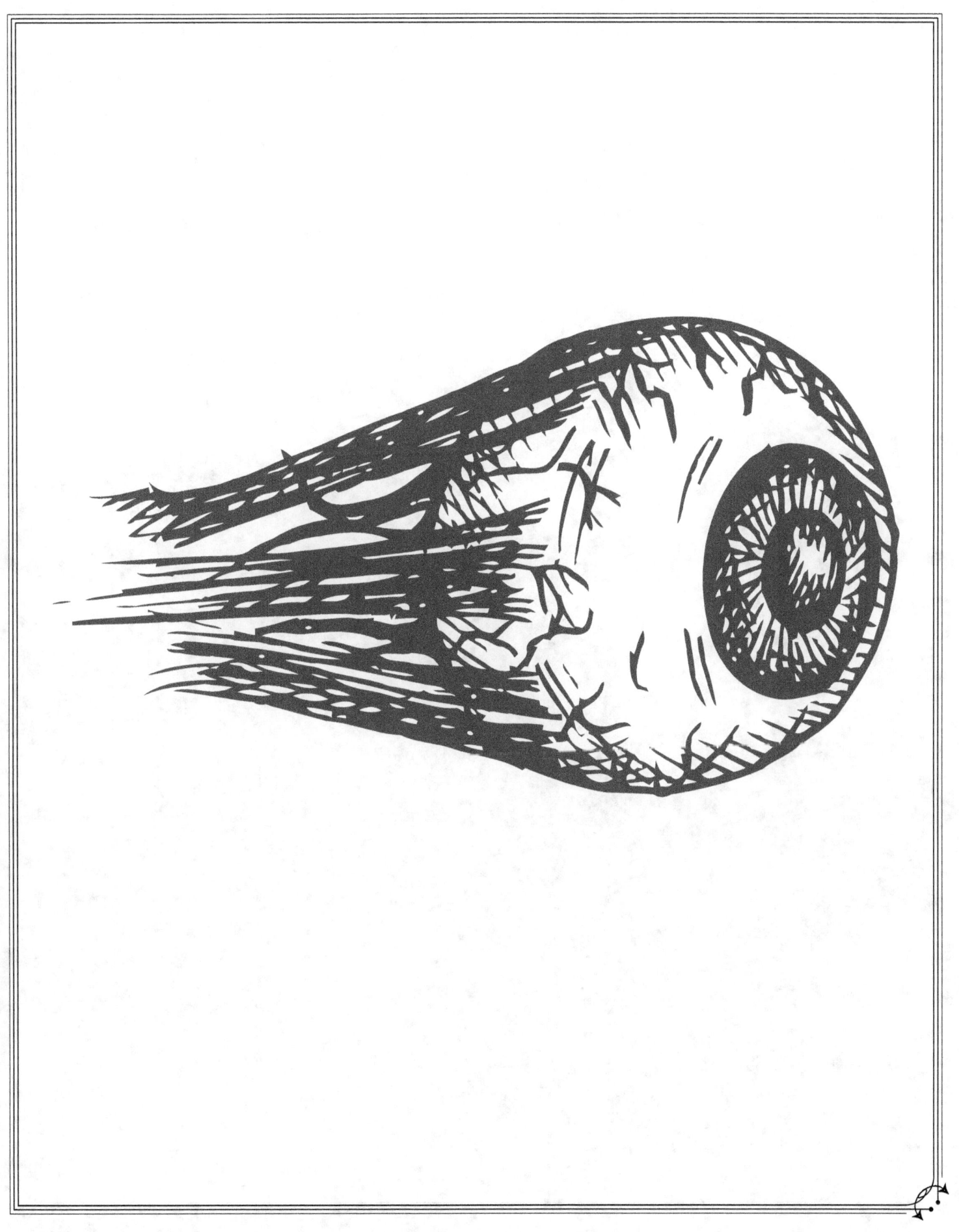

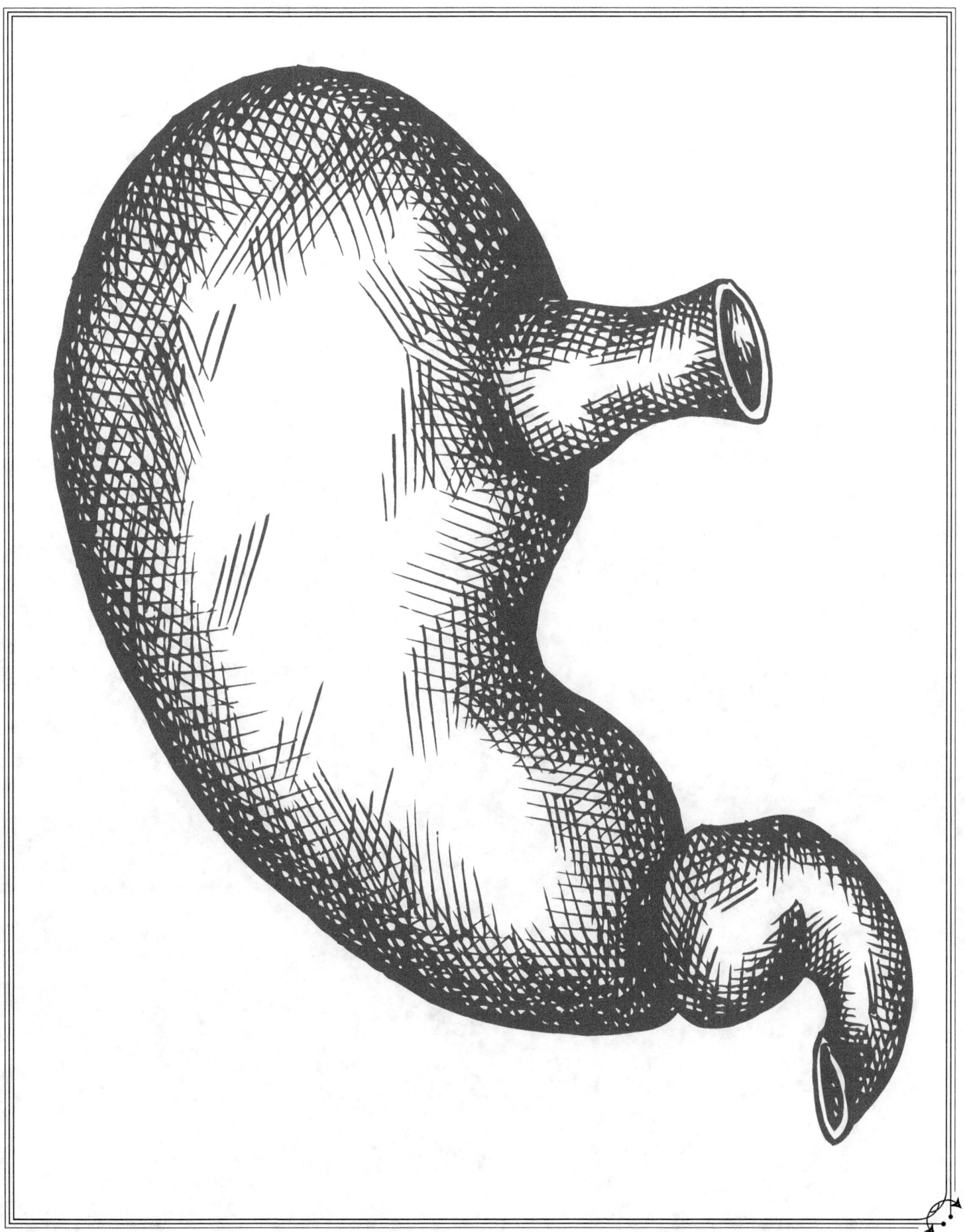

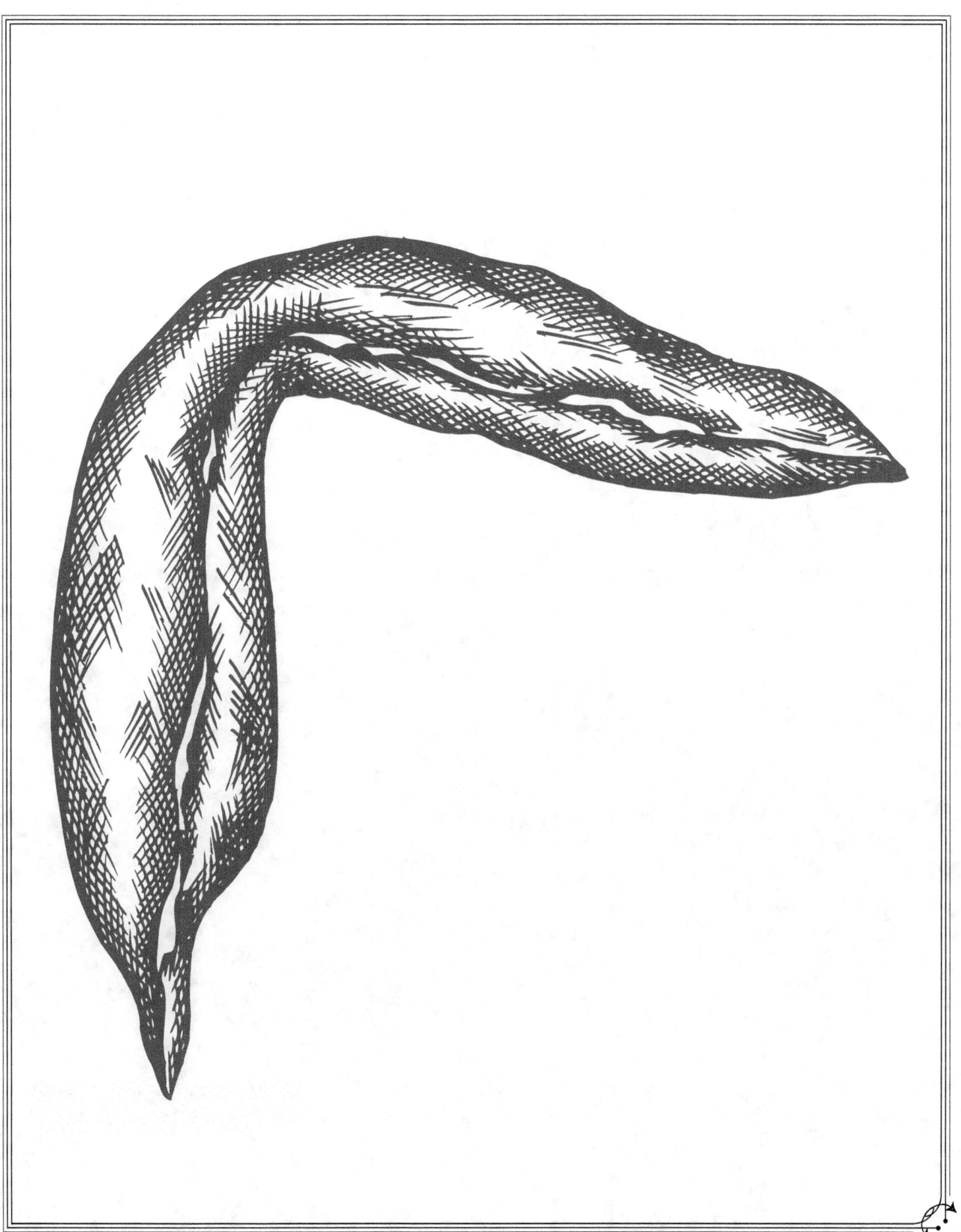

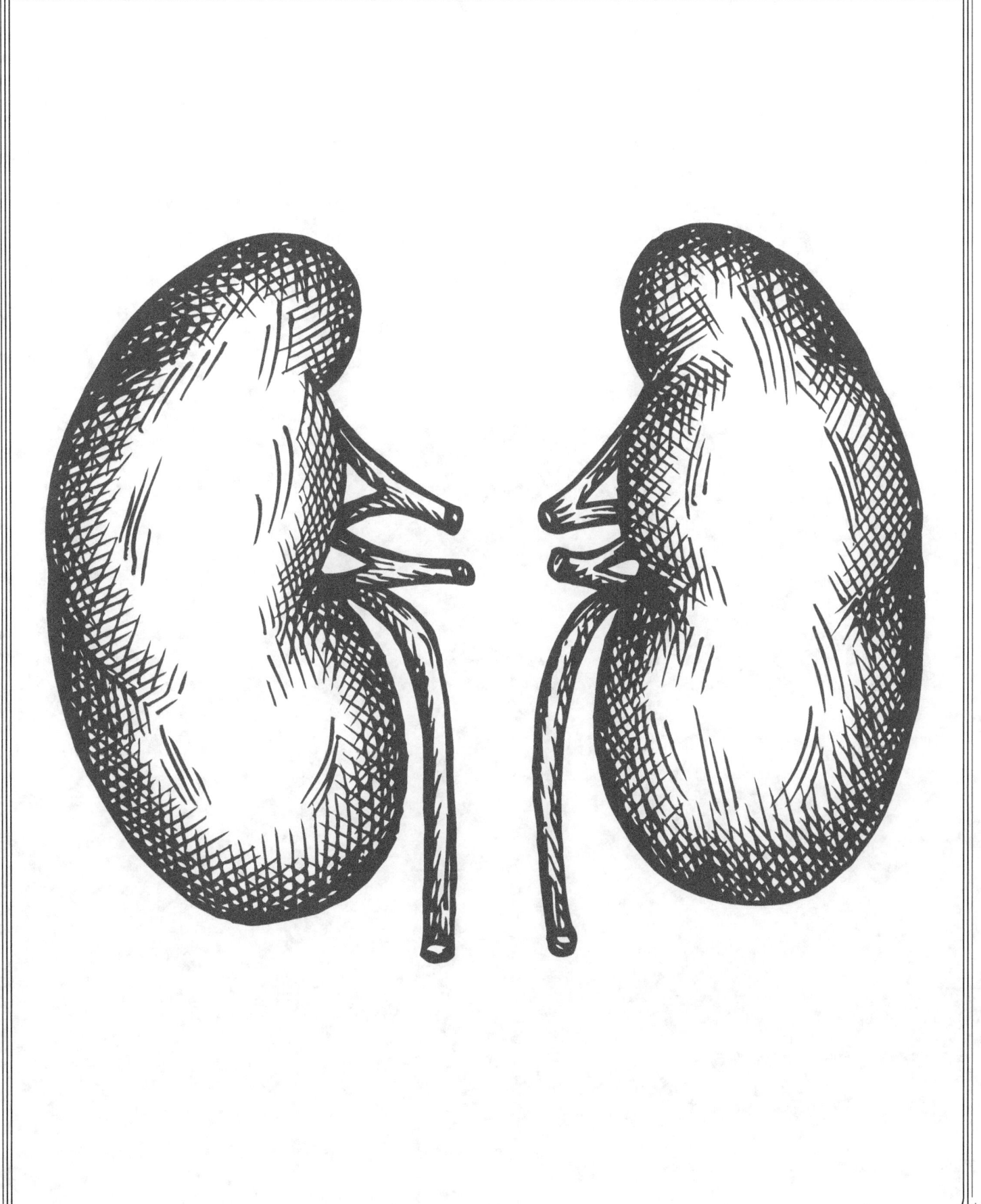

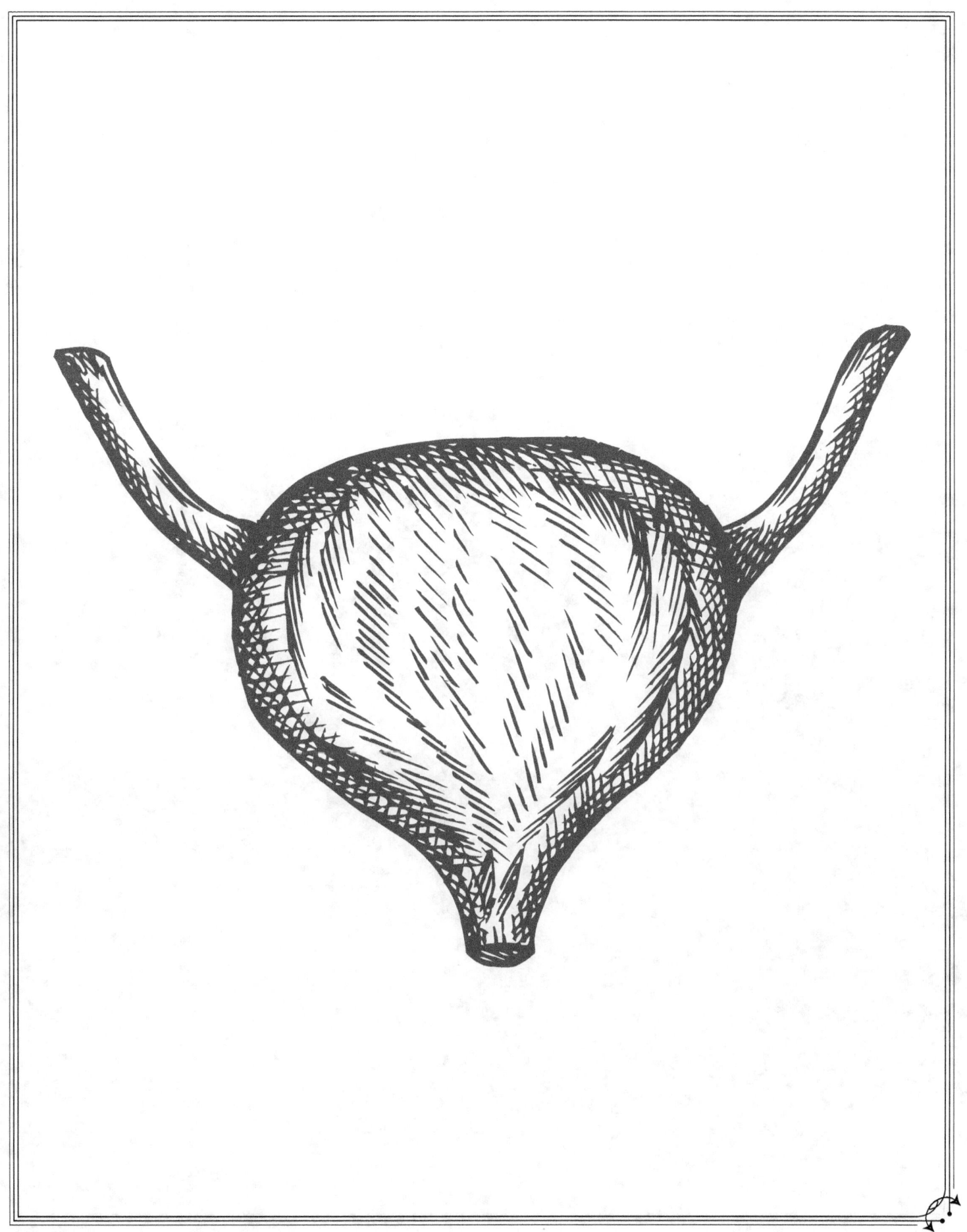

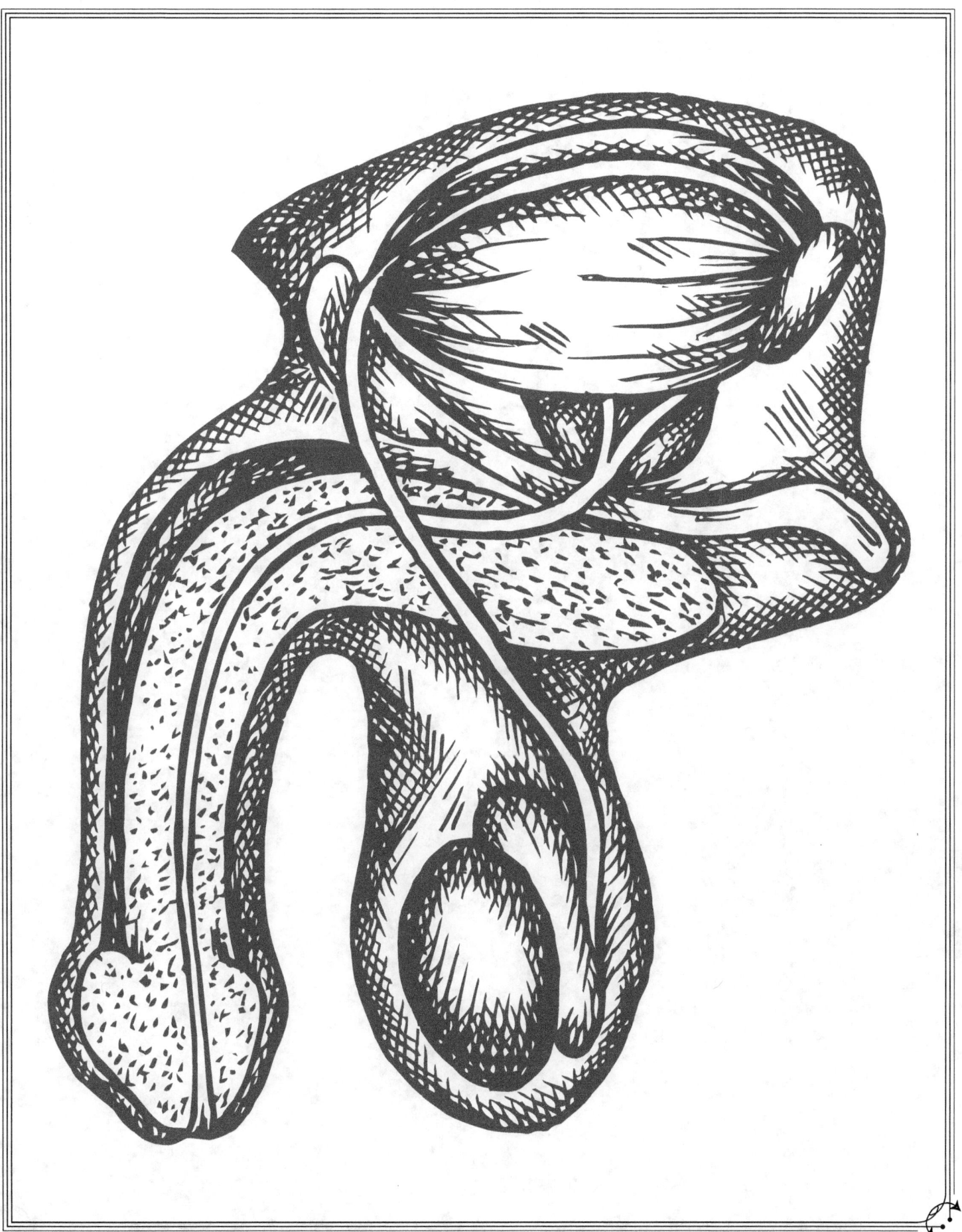

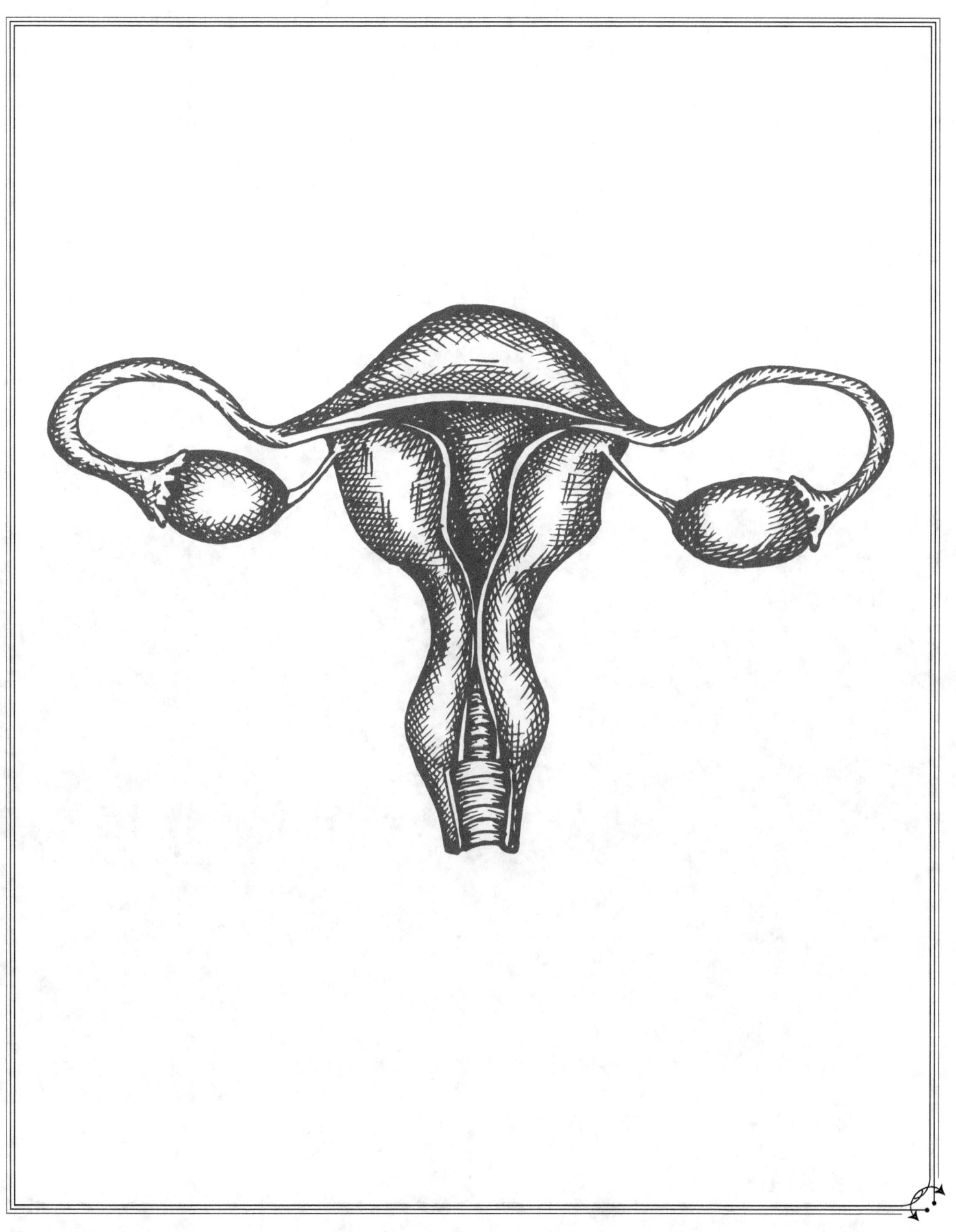

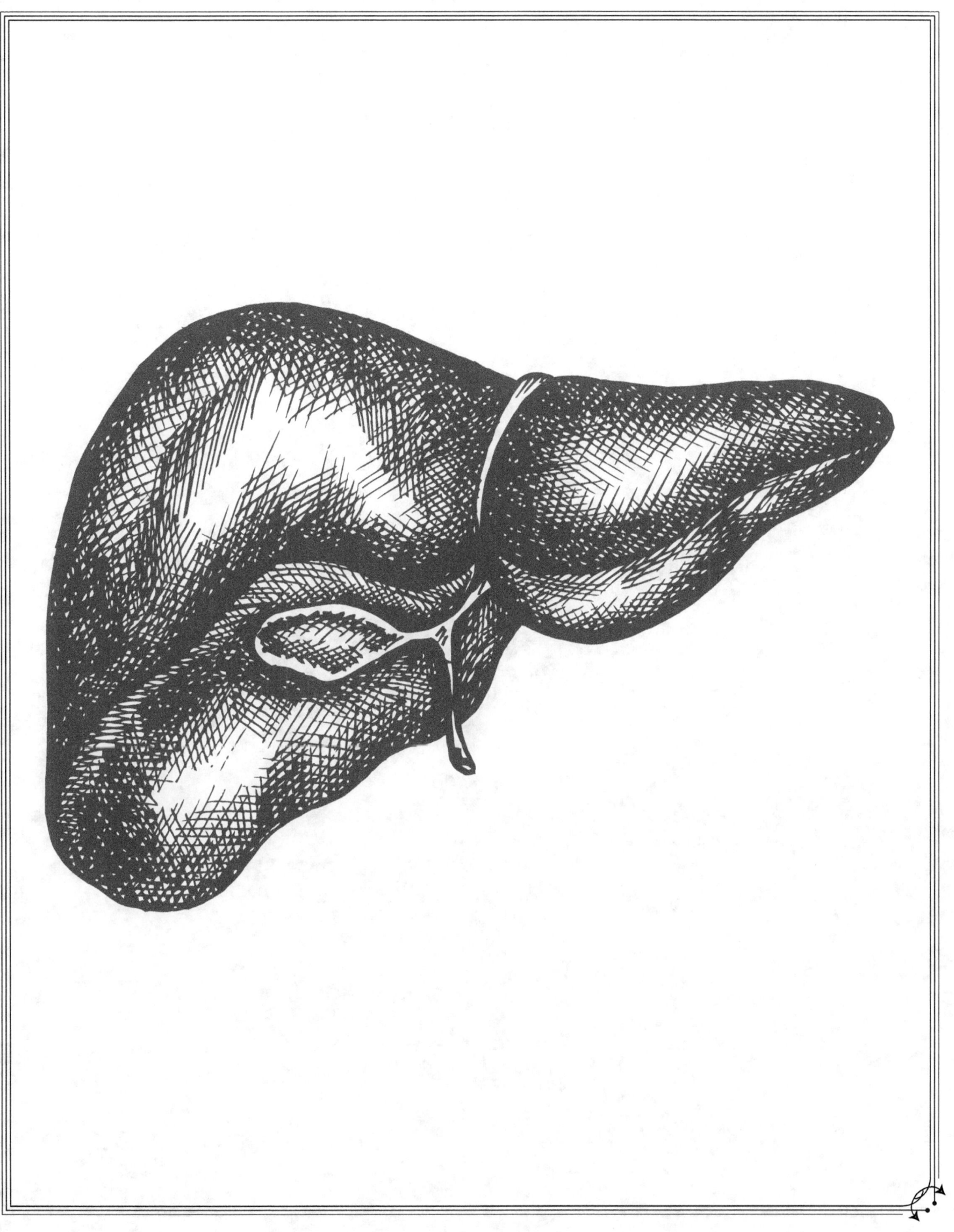

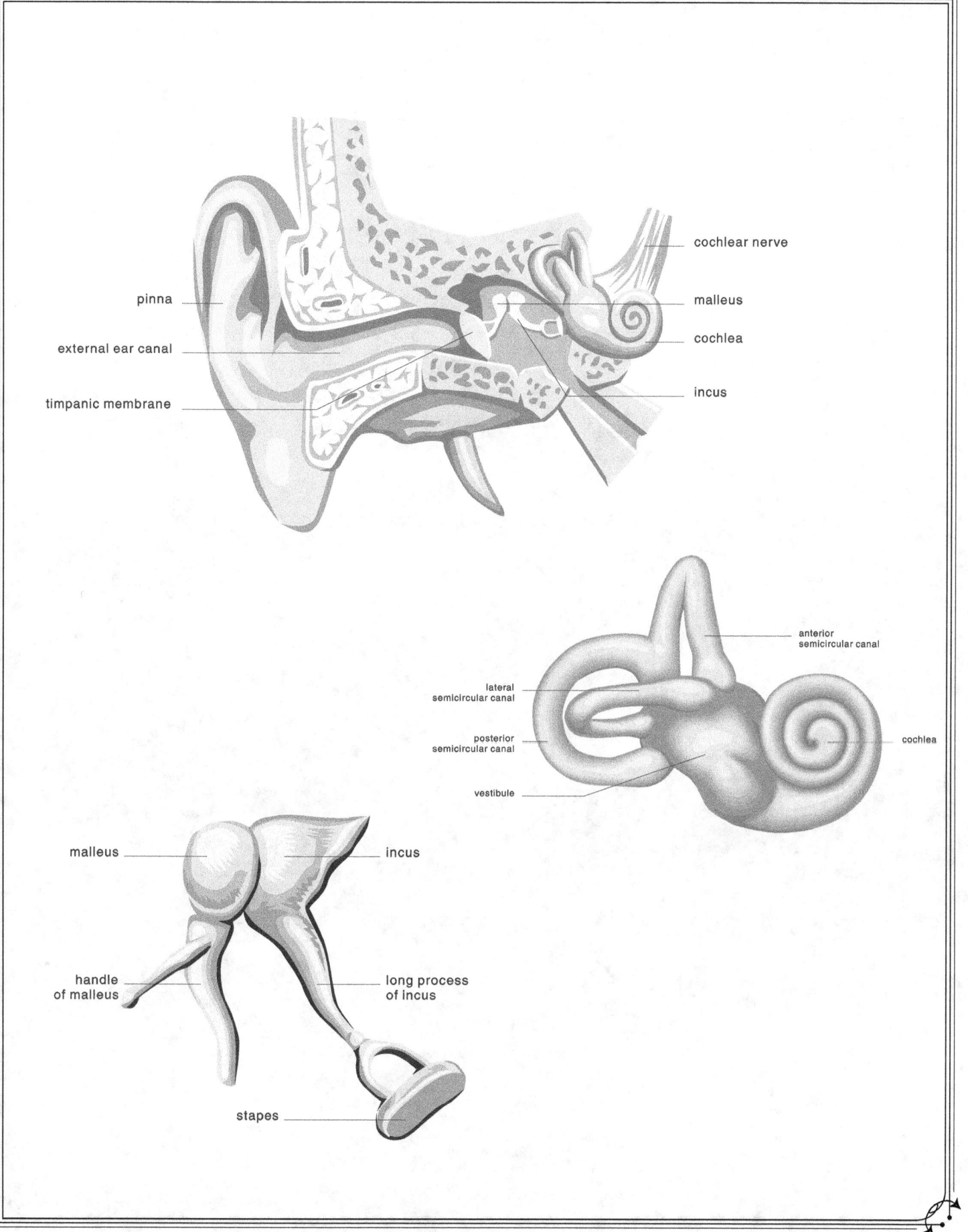

pinna

external ear canal

timpanic membrane

cochlear nerve

malleus

cochlea

incus

anterior
semicircular canal

lateral
semicircular canal

posterior
semicircular canal

vestibule

cochlea

malleus

incus

handle
of malleus

long process
of incus

stapes

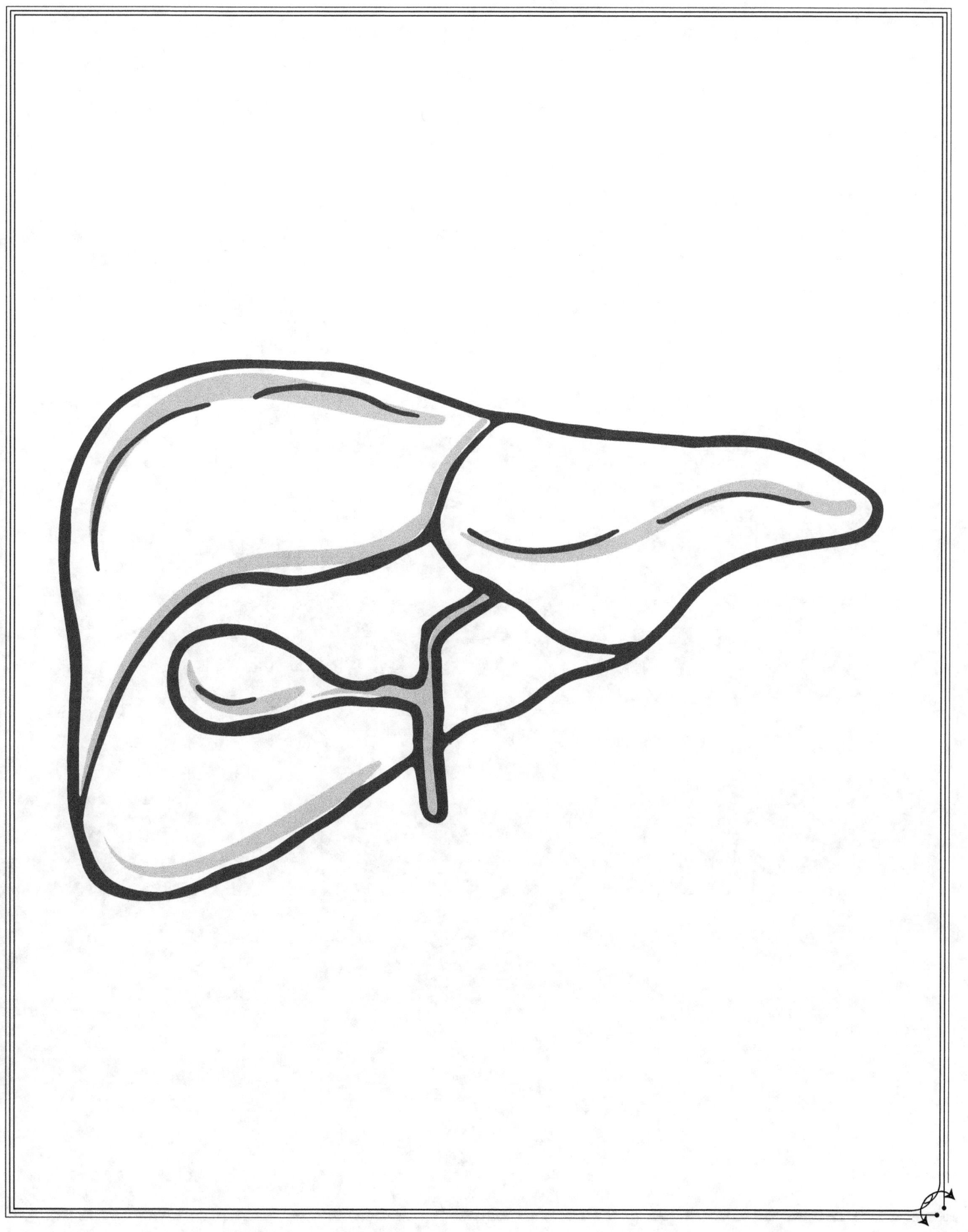

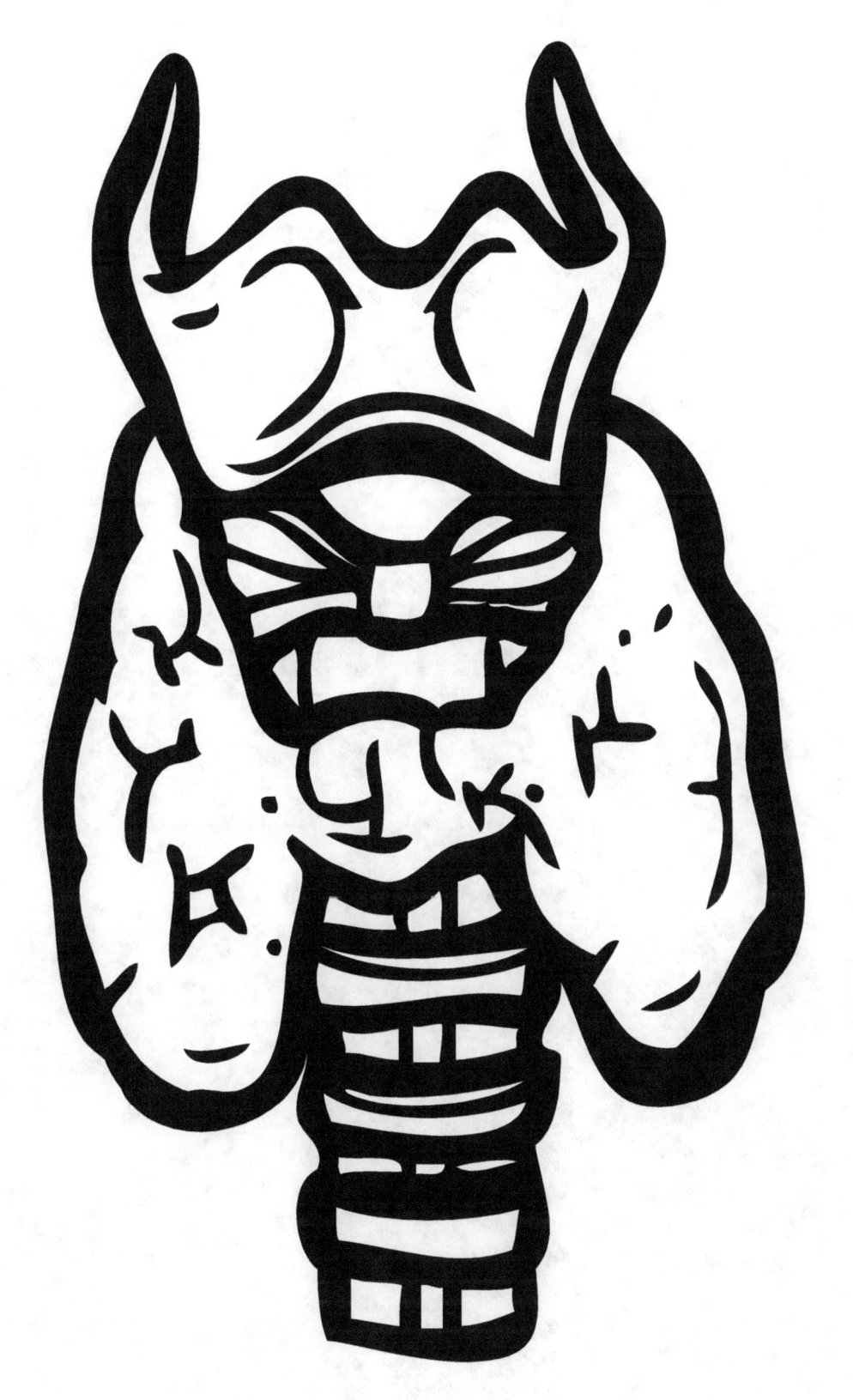

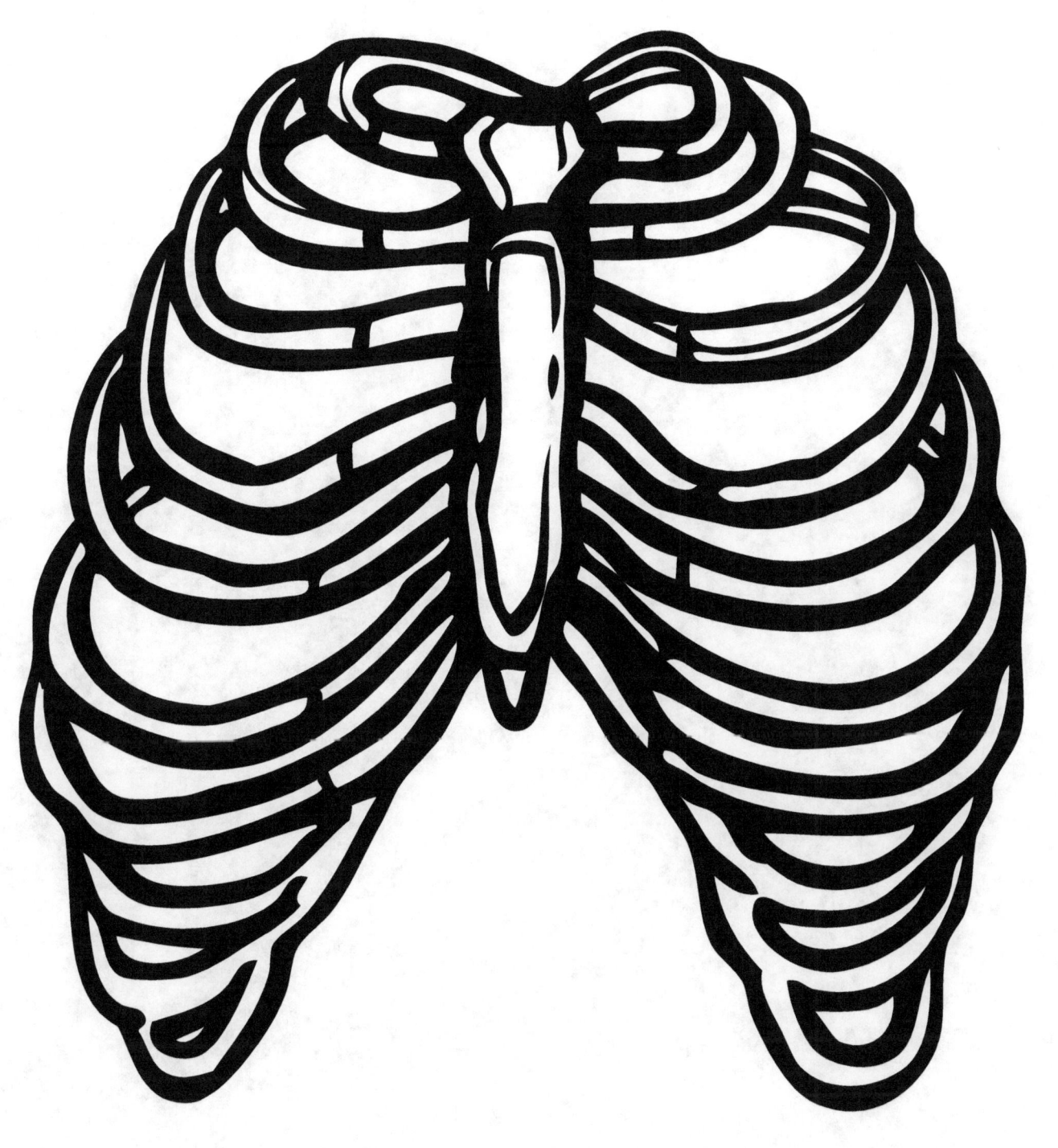

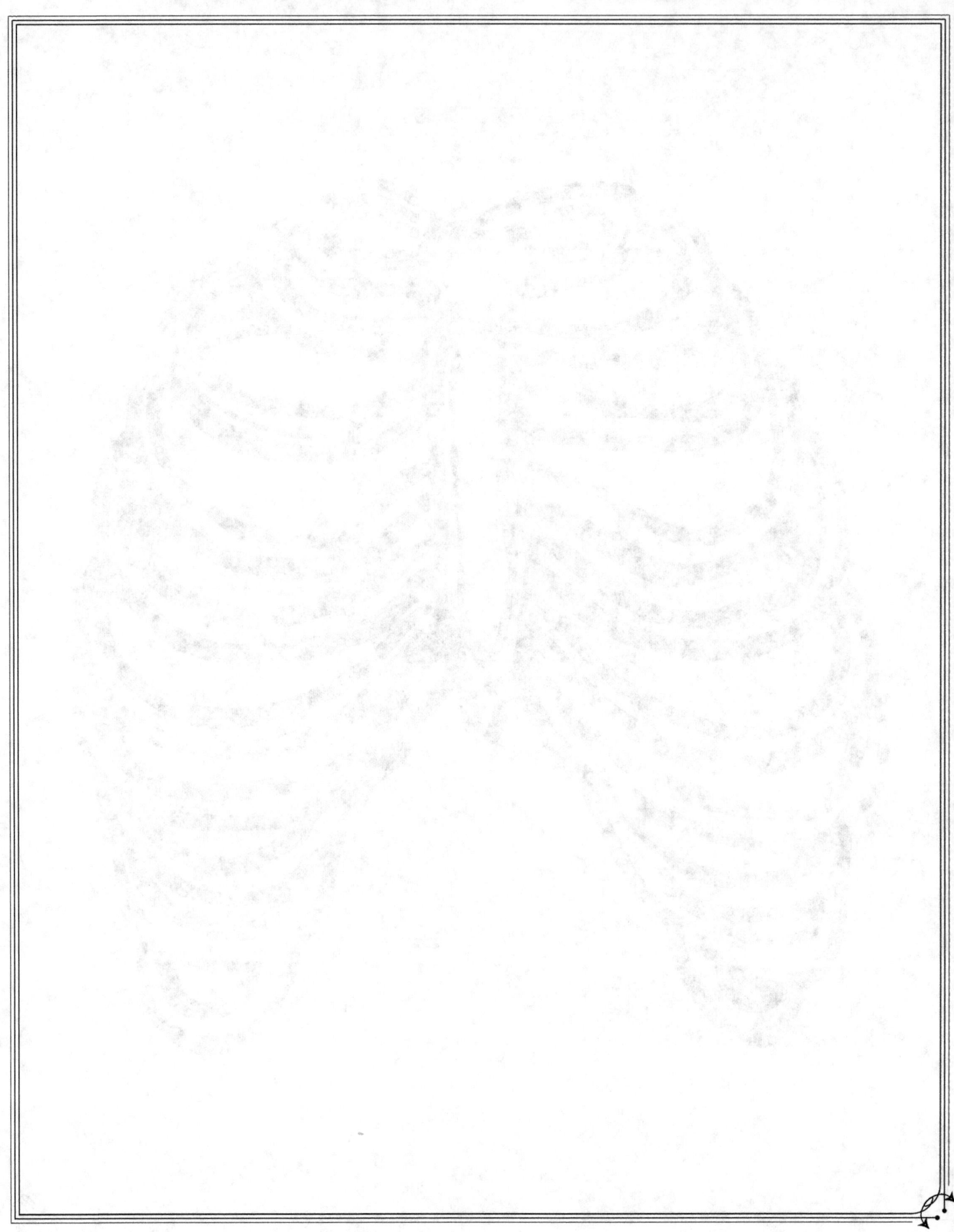

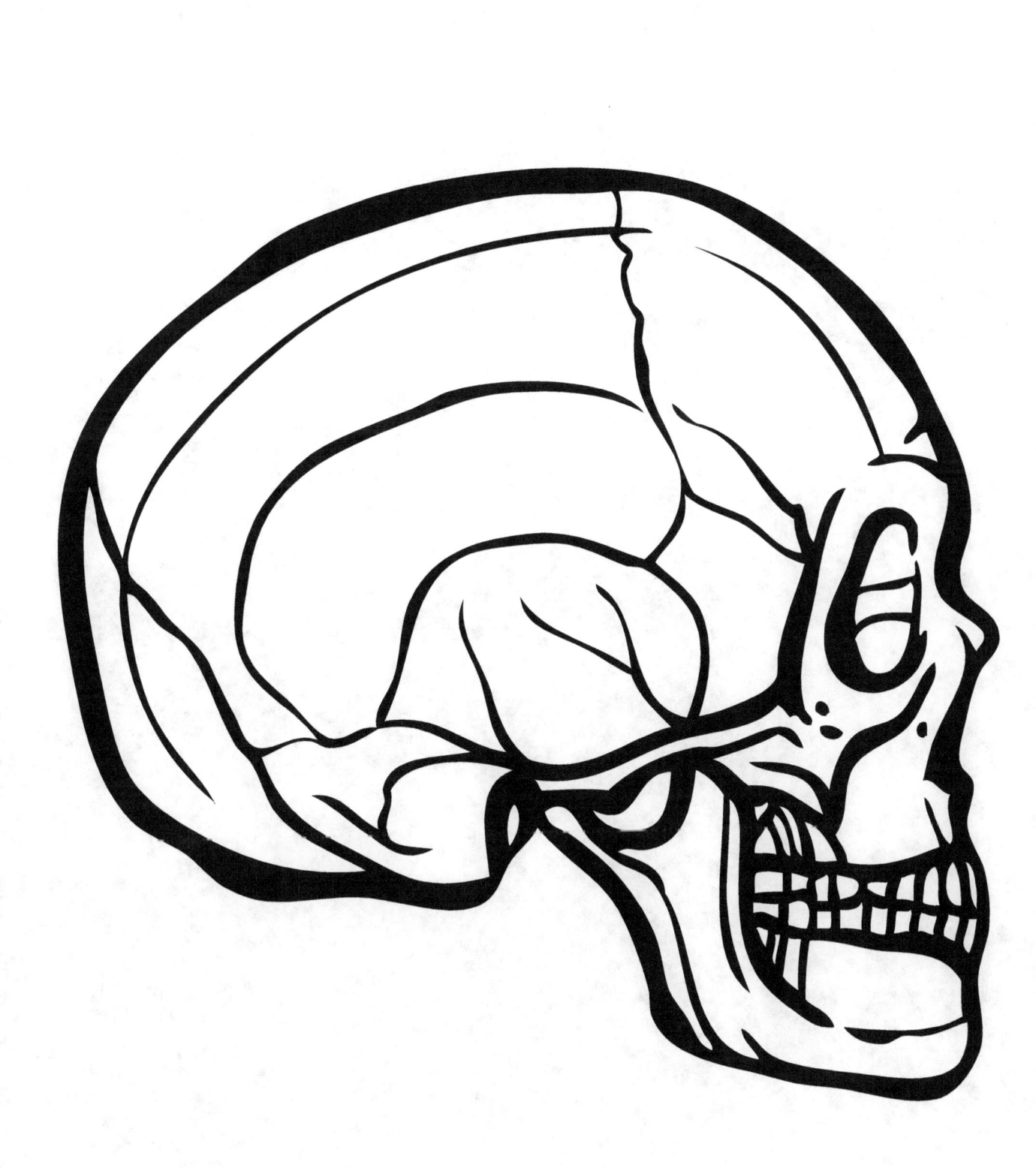

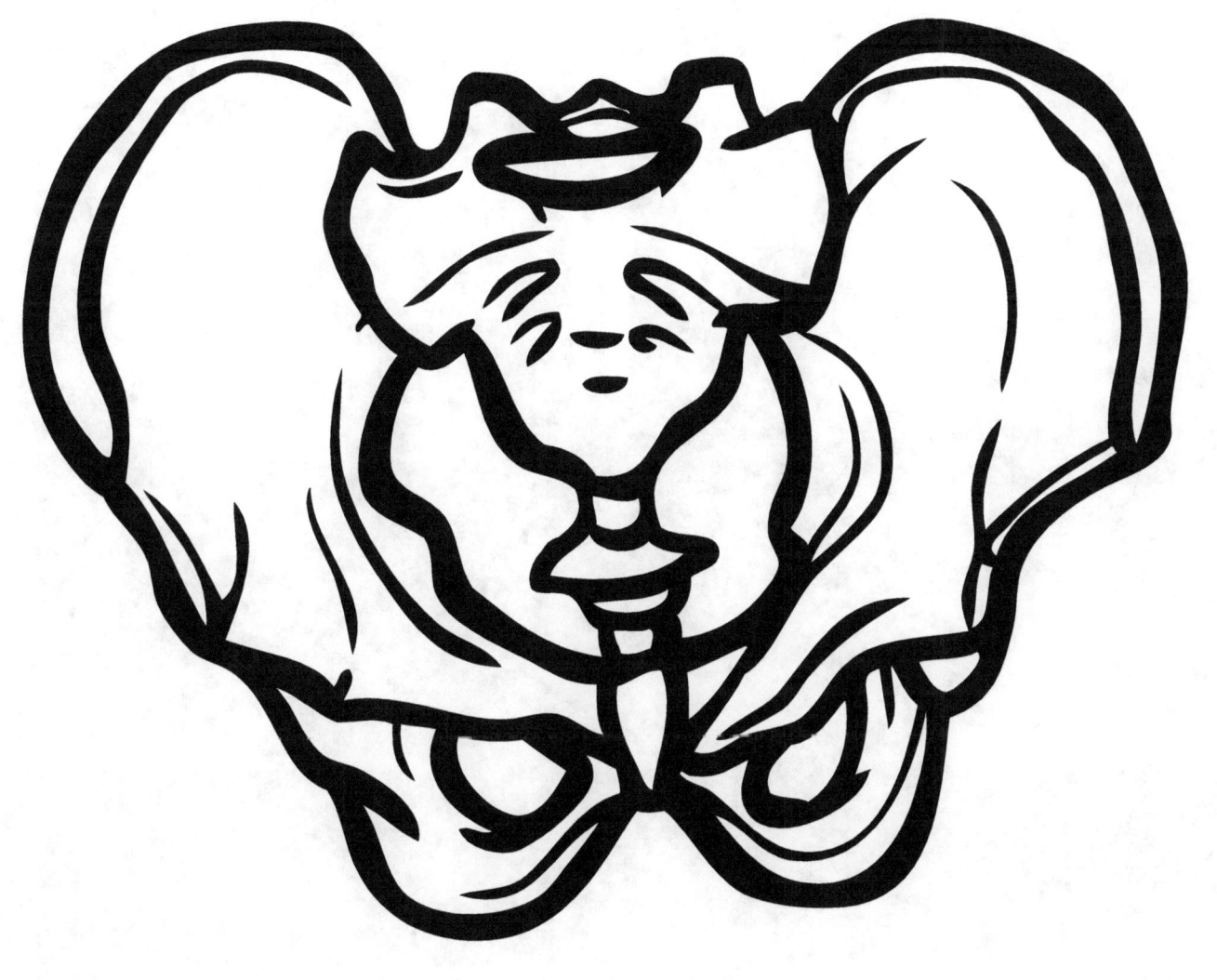

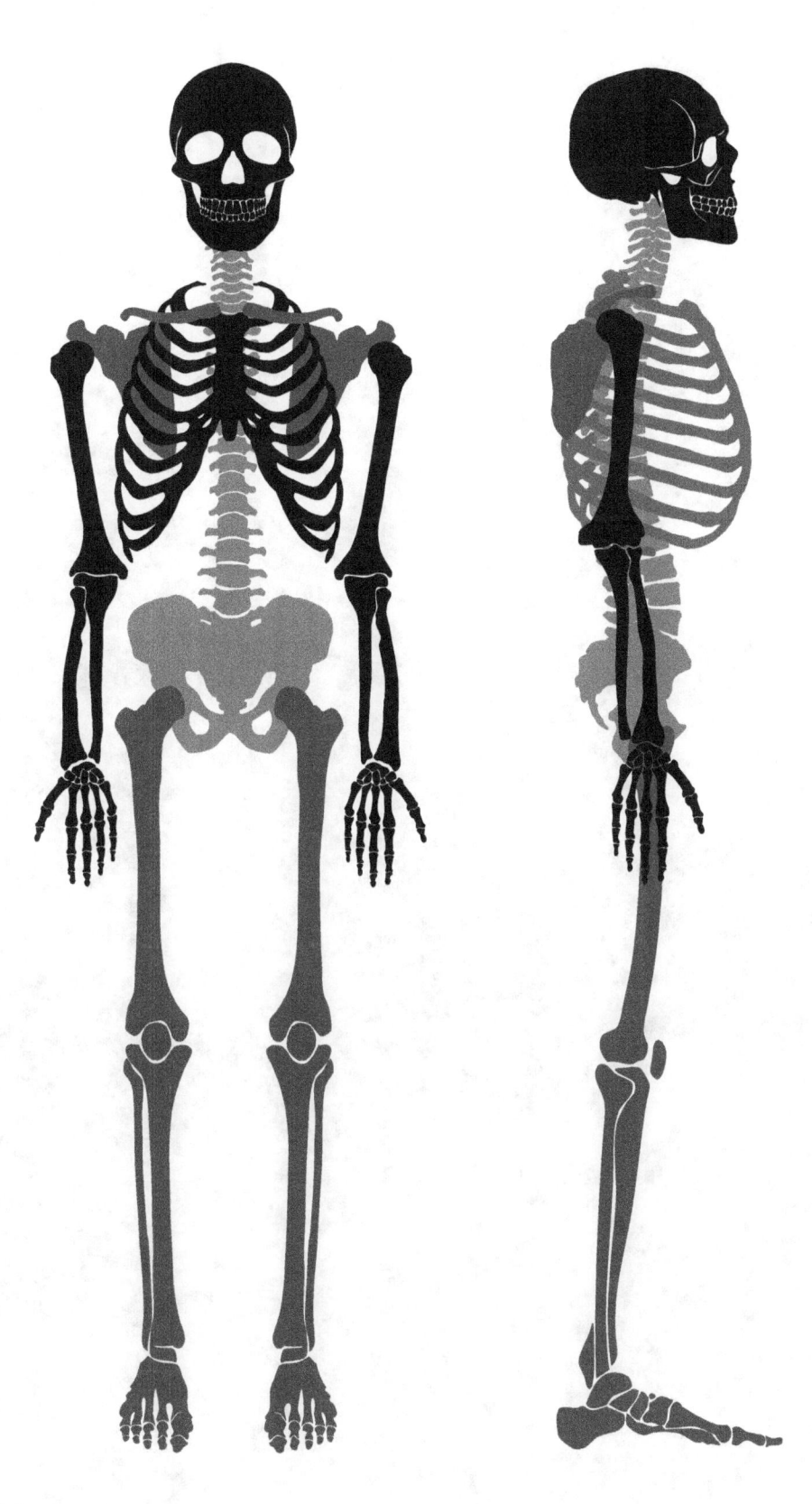

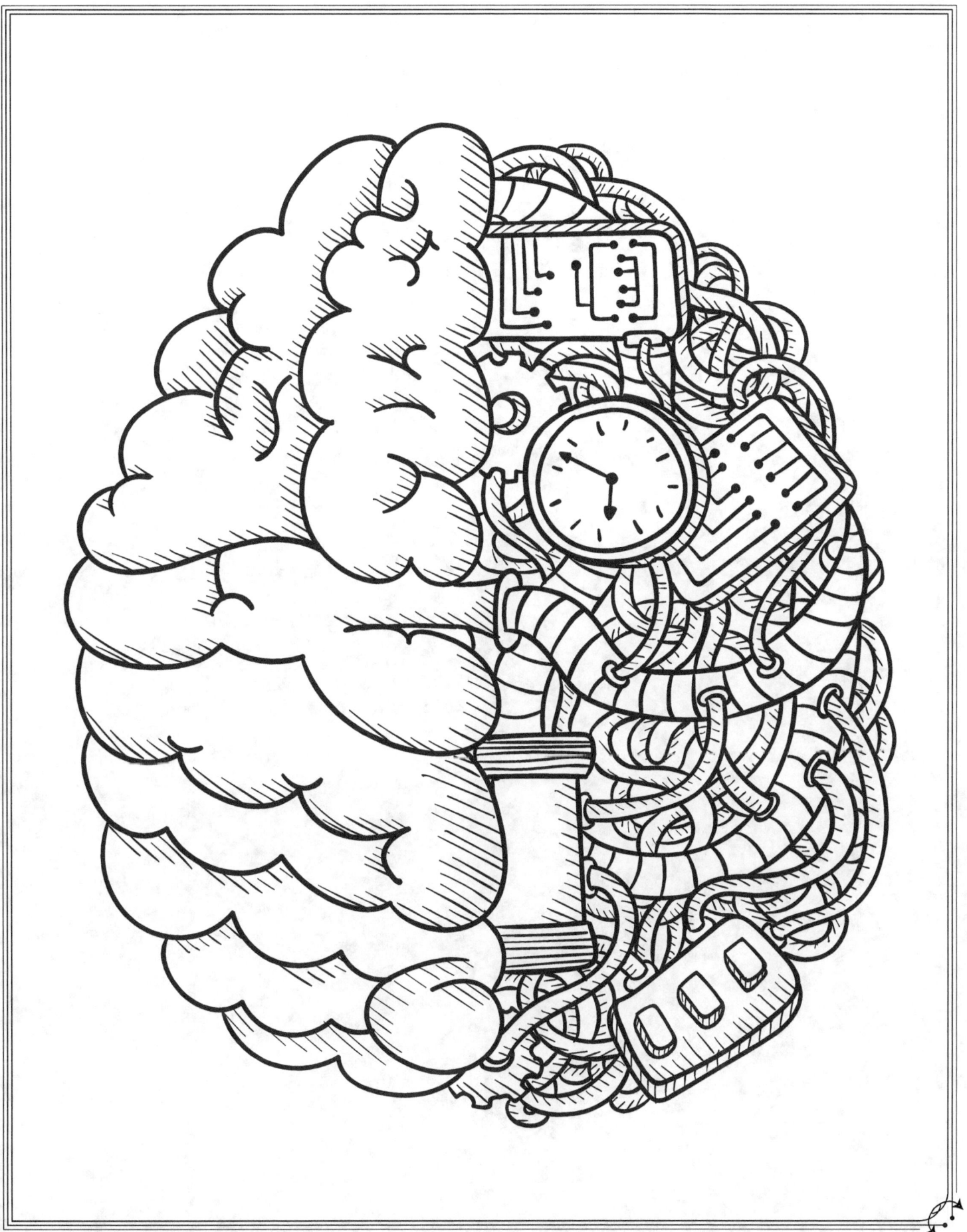

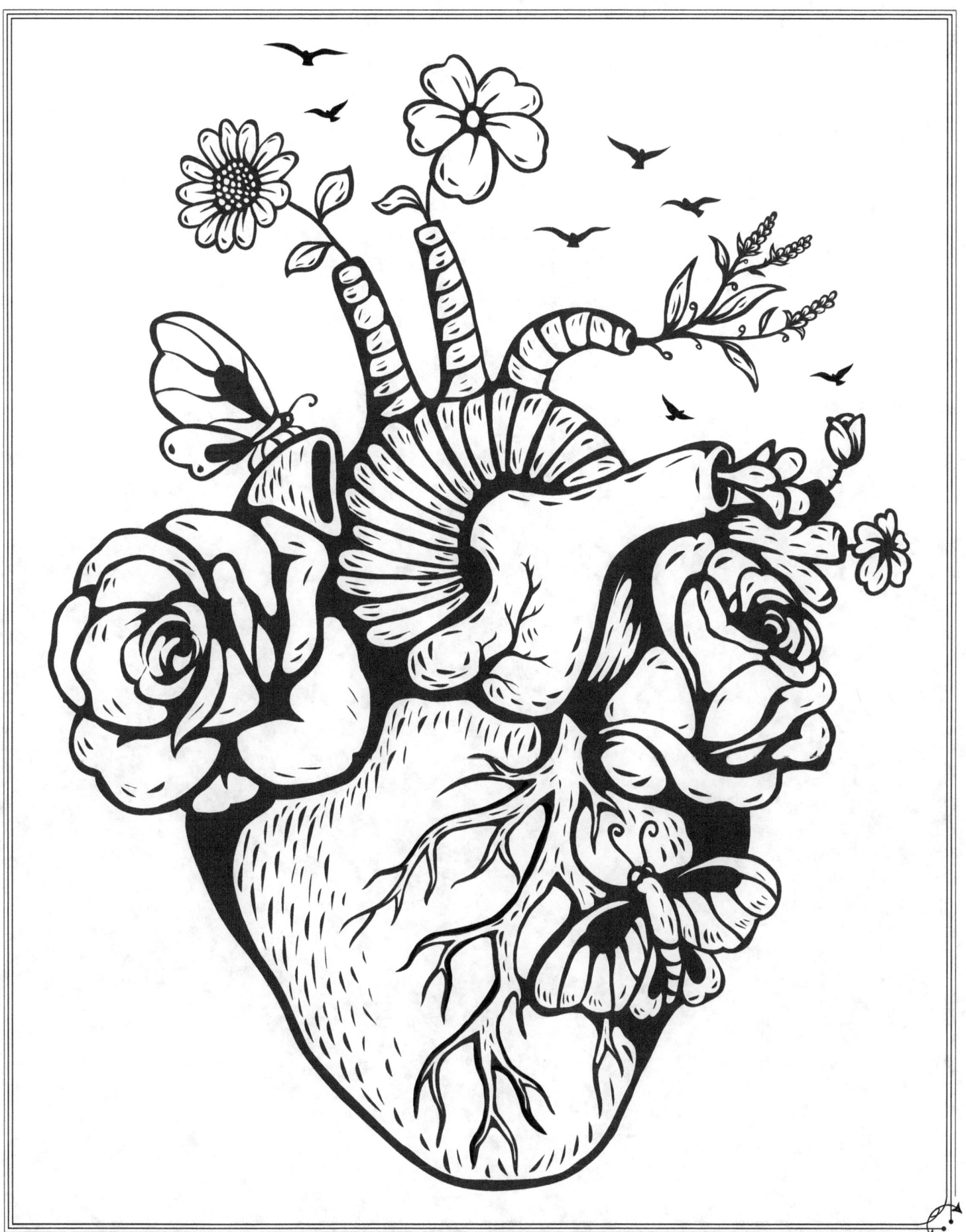

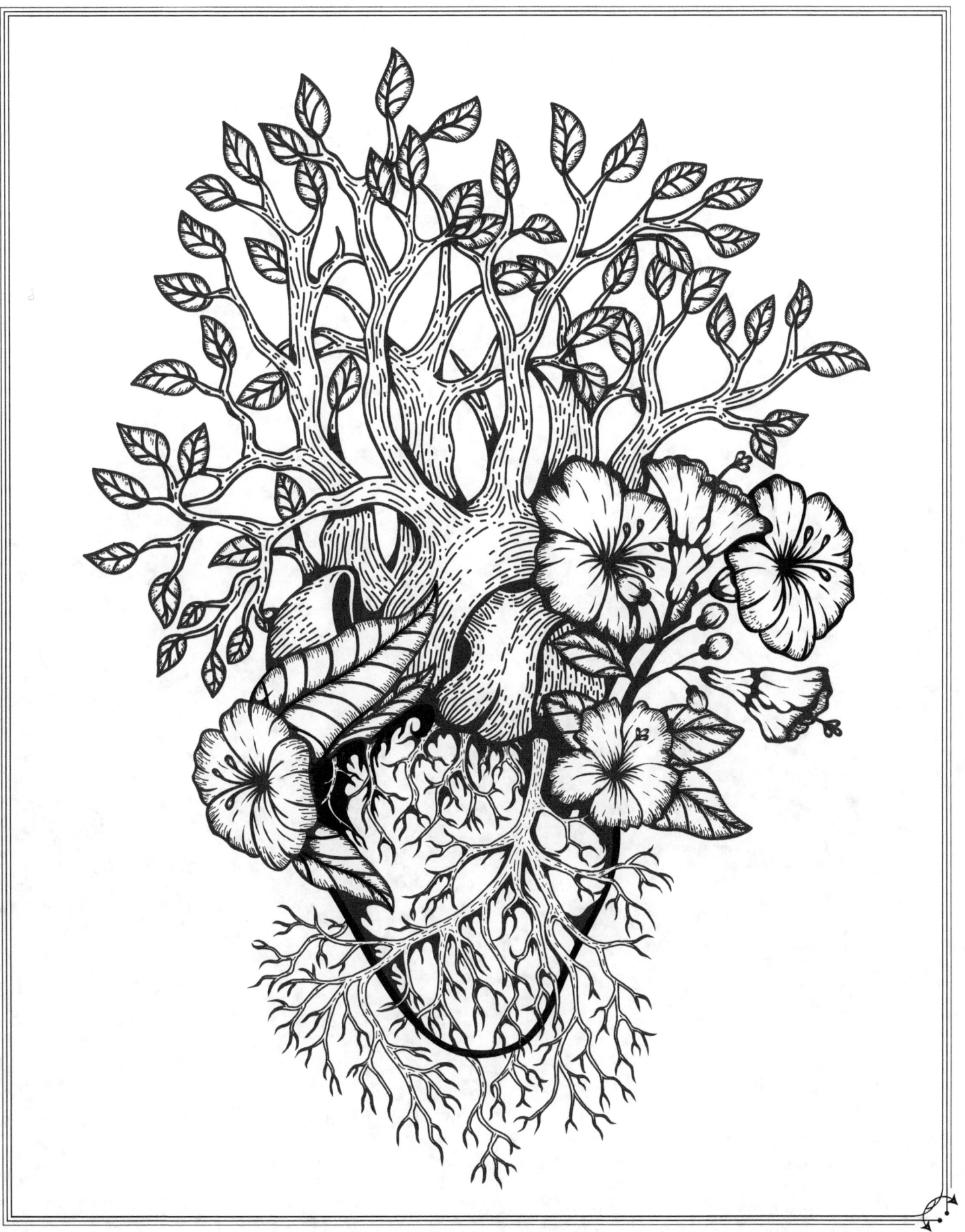